Potty Chair Training

Tips On How To Successfully Potty Train Your Child With Creativity And Confidence, Geared Toward Both Boys And Girls

Michele L. Valdez

Introducing the exclusive and captivating world of Michele L. Valdez. Immerse yourself in the timeless elegance and creativity that defines our brand. Experience the unparalleled craftsmanship and attention to detail that sets us apart. Discover the essence of sophistication and style with our exquisite collection.

Table of Contents

Preface

Are you prepared to go on a life-changing adventure with your child, putting the days of wearing diapers behind you and welcoming an era of self-reliance and confidence? Welcome to "Potty Chair Training" – a comprehensive guide to successfully navigating the exciting journey of potty training with a positive and enthusiastic approach.

Embark on a remarkable journey with us through the pages of this extraordinary book, where you will find an abundance of motivation, wisdom, and effective techniques to assist your child in overcoming the potty training obstacle. Right from the start, you'll experience the impact of storytelling as a powerful tool for capturing attention and inspiring others. With captivating stories of potty training triumphs and exciting adventures, your child will embark on an exhilarating journey towards success.

However, this book goes beyond storytelling and focuses on empowering parents with the necessary knowledge and confidence to provide unwavering support to their child throughout their journey. With professional guidance and tailored strategies, you will gain the skills to confidently navigate the challenges of the potty training journey with poise and determination. With "Potty Chair Training," you'll find guidance on how to navigate challenges and celebrate every little win, all while customizing the approach to suit your child's individuality.

One of the most captivating aspects of "Potty Chair Training" is its focus on engaging activities that bring joy and satisfaction to both you and your child. With a variety of engaging activities, these interactive exercises will turn potty training into an exciting journey. Through each activity, your child will develop a sense of self-assurance and self-reliance, establishing the groundwork for a lifetime of positive behaviors.

However, the most captivating aspect of "Potty Chair Training" is its empowering message. As you support your child during the process of potty training, you'll have the opportunity to witness their growth and development firsthand. Each day, they will become more confident, capable, and self-reliant. And as you commemorate their achievements together, you'll develop a connection that is more resilient than ever – a connection founded on trust, admiration, and shared comprehension.

So why hesitate? Come and join the countless parents who have already embarked on their own "Potty Adventures" and witness the profound impact it can have on your child's life. If you're new to potty training or in need of some new ideas to overcome a challenging obstacle, this book provides all the necessary tools for your success. Bid farewell to diapers and welcome a world filled with excitement - thanks to "Potty Chair Training."

Get your copy today and embark on your own potty training journey!

Introduction

Had enough of those never-ending diaper changes and messy accidents? Imagine a potty training experience that is completely stress-free for your child. Stop searching any longer! In "Potty Chair Training," Sarah Johnson, a renowned author and expert in parenting, presents a revolutionary method for potty training that is highly effective and brings joy to both children and parents.

With Sarah's effective techniques and expert advice, you'll uncover the keys to achieving stress-free and successful potty training. This comprehensive guide provides all the information you need to achieve potty training success, from selecting the perfect potty chair to overcoming common challenges.

Contained within are:

Detailed instructions, presented in a sequential manner: Follow Sarah's simple steps for introducing your child to the potty chair and building confidence with each successful milestone.

Effective Techniques for Motivating and Encouraging Your Child: Discover proven methods to inspire and uplift your child, fostering a strong sense of pride and accomplishment.

Helpful Suggestions for Resolving Issues: Conquer potty training setbacks with Sarah's expert guidance on managing accidents, resistance, and regression with poise and understanding.

Interactive Activities: Enhance the potty training experience by incorporating imaginative activities and games that will captivate your child's interest and maintain their enthusiasm for using the potty chair.

Support from Parents: Discover comfort and encouragement as Sarah tackles common worries and offers practical advice for confidently navigating the potty training journey.

By using "Potty Chair Training," you can bid farewell to diapers and welcome a world of independence and freedom for your child. Equip yourself with the knowledge and tools necessary to transform potty training into a positive and empowering journey for the entire family.

Say goodbye to the frustrations of potty training. Join the countless parents who have revolutionized their potty training journey with Sarah's exceptional guidance. Whether you're a beginner or facing challenges, "Potty Chair Training" is the ultimate resource to help you achieve potty training success.

Embark on the journey to a future without diapers. Get your hands on the "Potty Chair Training" book today!

C h a p t e r 1

Discover the Essential Factors to Consider When Selecting a Potty Chair or Potty Seat

Discover the remarkable distinction.

Discover the benefits of each method for Potty training!

Discover the remarkable distinction between a Potty Seat and Potty Chair, a question that may seem simple at first glance. Introducing our new and improved variations, now with even more exciting features! At our core, we are dedicated to delivering an abundance of high-quality information that empowers you to make the optimal decision for your loved ones.

Discover a wide variety of options to find the perfect choice for your entire family. Are you wondering, "Why should I use one instead of the other?"

Discover the art of effectively responding by:

- Gaining a deep understanding of your child's needs.

- Discover your child's passions and interests.

Discover the perfect solution that caters to your unique needs and desires. Consider various factors, such as what will truly enhance your family's lifestyle.

Discovering what truly suits your family is not always the same as what works for others. In fact, it all comes down to the unique desires and needs of your own family.

Discover the undeniable power of both methods as invaluable tools in successfully potty training your child. Discover the effortless and straightforward distinction between the Potty chair and the potty seat. The Potty chair stands alone as a separate entity, completely independent of the Potty. On the other hand, the potty seat is a stationary addition to your current Potty seat or can even replace it entirely, adapting and evolving alongside your child.

Discover the fascinating world of products available on the market, where positives and negatives intertwine to create a unique experience. Discover the multitude of options at your disposal, allowing you to make the optimal choice for your beloved family members.

Introducing the ultimate guide to the Potty chair: uncovering the experts, revealing the cons, and covering every aspect you need to know. Introducing our revolutionary Potty Seats - the ultimate solution for your child's potty training needs! These portable wonders are not only incredibly convenient, but they are also designed to be lightweight, allowing your little one to easily move it all by themselves. Say goodbye to the hassle and hello to independence with our innovative Potty Seats! Introducing our incredible selection of Potty Chairs, designed to make potty training an absolute delight! Discover a world of tempting and fun shapes, available in a variety of sizes that are perfect for your little one. And that's not all - some of our Potty Chairs even come with delightful musical features, adding an extra touch of joy to the potty training journey. Say goodbye to boring potty chairs and say hello to a world of excitement and convenience!

Discover a world of whimsical character types and captivating designs that will bring joy and excitement to your little one's potty seat. Discover the power of visual motivation for your child! With captivating designs that are sure to inspire, you can unlock their full potential. Studies show that children of this age learn best when they are visually stimulated. Don't miss out on this incredible opportunity to enhance your child's learning experience!

Introducing the ultimate solution for parents whose children are captivated by pets or their favorite characters - behold the incredible viewing experience right from the comfort of their seat! This extraordinary addition will provide the extra push your child needs to take their development to the next level.

Introducing our versatile collection of seats, designed to cater to your every need. Take, for instance, our exquisite throne themed chair, fit for a little prince or princess like yours. Its timeless design seamlessly blends with any décor, making it the perfect addition to your home. Introducing our incredible Potty seats, the ultimate solution for your child's comfort and growth! Not only do these seats provide a secure and comfortable place for your little one to do their business, but they also double as a rocking seat once they outgrow the potty training phase. It's the perfect investment that will grow with your child and provide endless hours of fun and relaxation. Don't miss out on this versatile and innovative product!

Introducing our exquisite collection of wooden Potty chairs, designed with utmost care and attention to detail. Each chair comes complete with a convenient wall paper and publication holder, providing you with the ultimate in functionality and style. And the best part? The holder can be easily removed, giving you the freedom to customize your Potty chair to suit your unique taste and preferences. Experience the perfect blend of practicality and elegance with our wooden Potty chairs.

Introducing our revolutionary Potty Seats! Designed with your child in mind, these child-size seats ensure that their little feet can easily reach the bottom, promoting a more natural and comfortable potty position. Say goodbye to discomfort and hello to impressive eliminations!

Discover the empowering benefits of Potty Seats, unlocking a world of independence for your little one. Experience the exciting journey of childhood development as your little ones explore their boundaries and strive for independence. With our innovative Potty chair, they can confidently navigate this stage without the need for constant assistance.

Discover the Ultimate Guide to Selecting the Perfect Potty Chair!

Embark on a quest to find the ultimate Potty chair and prepare to be dazzled by a myriad of options, each boasting unique choices, stylish designs, and a range of sizes. Introducing our incredible selection of Potty chairs! Experience the convenience and versatility of our one-piece designs or explore the endless possibilities of our multifunctional Potty chairs. Whether you're at home or on the go, our Potty chairs have got you covered. Say goodbye to the hassle of traveling with toddlers - our travel Potty chair is here to make your journeys a breeze.

Discover the ultimate solution for all your Potty chair needs!

Discover the 5 Essential Potty Chair Variations:

- *Introducing the revolutionary One Piece Potty Chair* - the ultimate solution for your little one's potty training journey. With its innovative design and unparalleled comfort, this potty chair is a game-changer. Say goodbye to messy accidents and hello to stress-free potty time. Trust the

- *Introducing our innovative Removable Chamber* - the perfect solution for all your needs.

- *Introducing our revolutionary Multi-function Potty Chairs!*

- *Introducing the ultimate bathroom chair.*

- *Introducing the ultimate solution for on-the-go potty needs* - the Travel Potty Chair & Seats! Say goodbye to inconvenient bathroom breaks and hello to hassle-free potty time. Whether you're embarking on a road trip or exploring new destinations, our Travel Potty Chair & Seats are here to make your life easier.

Experience the elegance of One Piece Design.

Introducing the Pros of our product:

- Experience simplicity and convenience like never before with our sleek and portable design.

- Introducing our low-profile design - perfect for your little one to effortlessly hop on and off the potty. Not only that, but it also promotes a higher, more natural squatting position for a comfortable potty experience.

- Experience the ultimate convenience with our light-weight and compact design.

- Discover the unbeatable affordability.

- Introducing our latest product innovation: a design that prioritizes your safety and comfort. Say goodbye to pinching and sharp edges with our meticulously crafted product. Experience a new level of smoothness and elegance like never before.

Introducing the Potty chair, the perfect solution for all your potty training needs. However, one small drawback is that you need to subject the complete Potty chair in the Potty. But don't worry, with its innovative design and easy-to-use features, the Potty chair will make potty training a breeze for both you and your little one.

- Introducing our revolutionary low-profile and lightweight design! Say goodbye to those pesky tripping hazards, like toys on the floor. With our product, your toddler will be able to move freely and safely, without any unexpected tumbles.

- Introducing our perfectly sized product, designed with the utmost care to cater to the needs of smaller children. However, please note that it may not be suitable for much bigger children.

- Introducing the revolutionary Removable Chamber Chair! Experience the ultimate convenience and effortless tidying with this innovative piece of furniture. Say goodbye to the hassle of cleaning around chair legs and corners. With its removable chamber, tidying up has never been easier. Simply detach the chamber, clean it, and reattach it in a breeze. No more struggling to reach those hard-to-clean areas! The Removable Chamber

Introducing our incredible range of models, each one thoughtfully designed to include convenient lids. Say goodbye to spills and hello to hassle-free storage!

Introducing the incredible portable option:

a smaller version that you can take with you wherever you go!

Introducing the most popular and widely used potty chairs!

Discover the downsides:

Experience potential discomfort with pinching of your child's delicate bottom or thighs.

Note that many models lack portability, limiting their convenience.

Introducing our revolutionary Multifunctional Potty Chairs! Experience the ultimate convenience with our 2-in-1 Design that not only provides a comfortable potty seat but also a removable potty seat. Say goodbye to the hassle of constantly switching between seats - our innovative design has got you covered!

Introducing our revolutionary 3-in-1 Design! This incredible product combines the functionality of a potty chair, potty chair, and step stool all in one. Say goodbye to clutter and hello to convenience with our innovative solution.

Introducing our innovative 4-in-1 Design! This incredible product combines a potty chair, step stool, and storage compartments all in one. Say goodbye to clutter and hello to convenience! With ample space for playthings, books, and other rewards, our versatile design is perfect for any child's needs. Experience the ultimate in functionality and organization with our 4-in-1 Design.

Experience a seamless transition to the world of potty training with our easy-to-use system.

Introducing the Cons:

Experience the grandeur of its size and presence.

Introducing our latest innovation: a product that combines convenience and portability like never before. Say goodbye to the hassle of lugging around heavy equipment. Our revolutionary design ensures that you can take it with you wherever you go, effortlessly. Experience the

Introducing our premium Potty chairs, designed to elevate your child's potty training experience. While they may be priced slightly higher than traditional options, rest assured that the quality and features of our Potty chairs are worth every penny. Invest in your child's comfort and convenience with our top-of-the-line Potty chairs.

Introducing our exclusive collection of limited edition designs.

Introducing the Revolutionary Potty Chairs! Experience the ultimate convenience with our state-of-the-art Potty

Chairs. Say goodbye to messy clean-ups and hello to a hassle-free potty training journey. With our innovative design, your little one will feel like they're using the real potty, making the transition seamless and comfortable. Don't miss out on this game-changing solution!

Discover the only downside to this amazing product: • Some children may find the potty a bit overwhelming, as their feet may dangle, making it difficult for them to fully relax.

Discover the potential impact on your child's independence as they receive the necessary assistance.

Discover the ultimate solution for adult use - a product that must be removed to fully indulge in its benefits.

Introducing the Ultimate Travel Potty Chairs!

Introducing the ultimate solution for on-the-go potty needs - the Travel Potty Chair and Travel Potty Seats! Say goodbye to inconvenient bathroom breaks and hello to hassle-free travel with our innovative portable potty solutions. Whether you're embarking on a road trip, camping adventure, or simply need a reliable potty option for your little one.

Experience the ultimate convenience.

Experience the ultimate in security and comfort for your child.

Introducing our revolutionary product:

Sanitary, the ultimate solution for all your hygiene needs. Say goodbye to germs and hello to cleanliness with Sanitary.

Introducing the ultimate life saver! Experience the freedom of spontaneous outings without worrying about potty breaks for your little ones. Say goodbye to the stress of planning ahead while enjoying a night out at the pub.

Discover the downsides:

• Not crafted for everyday use.

• Comes with an extra cost.

Introducing the Ultimate Potty Solution: Potty Chair and Potty Seats!

Discover the ultimate essential for stress-free potty training: the Potty. While there are countless commercial products available, nothing compares to the simplicity and effectiveness of this must-have item. Say goodbye to the struggles and hello to success with the Potty. Introducing the all-new commercial brands that will revolutionize the way small children enjoy their meals! Gone are the days of simple containers and dishes. Now, experience the ultimate comfort and vibrant colors that will ignite your child's motivation like never before. Upgrade their mealtime experience with our exciting range of commercial brands.

Introducing the two fundamental varieties of commercial potties:

Introducing the revolutionary Potty Chair - the perfect solution for your little one's potty training journey. Say goodbye to messy accidents and hello to stress-free potty time! With its ergonomic design and comfortable

Introducing our revolutionary self-contained models that elegantly rest on the floor. Discover the incredible power of our products to enhance children's sense of security and captivate their curiosity, even when they are on their own. Experience the magic of our low-height designs! Introducing the ultimate solution for hassle-free bathroom breaks - our innovative detachable dish! Say goodbye to the inconvenience of transporting a full potty - simply detach the dish, empty it, and give it a quick rinse after each use. Experience the freedom and ease you deserve with our game-changing design. Introducing the perfect solution for little ones struggling with the transition from their beloved potty seat to the standard potty! Say goodbye to potty training woes with our innovative product.

Introducing our revolutionary Potty Seats!

Introducing our innovative solution: specially designed to fit snugly around the seat of a standard Potty, our product creates a secure and smaller space, ensuring that children stay safe and avoid any accidental falls. Experience the joy of growing up with the Potty, just like older siblings and parents! While some little ones simply love the sensation, we understand that many children may feel a bit apprehensive about the height. But fear not, for we have the perfect solution! Experience the thrilling challenge of ascending to new heights, where every step is a testament to your determination. Embrace the exhilaration of conquering obstacles, knowing that each moment is an opportunity for growth. Let the fear of a potential fall fuel your drive to push beyond your limits and achieve greatness. With every training session, you'll not only strengthen your body but also cultivate a resilient mindset. Embrace the adventure that awaits as you embark on this transformative journey.

Introducing an array of impressive features for your consideration:

- Introducing the remarkable feature of stableness! Our Potty seat is designed with a wider bottom and a top that is at least as wide, ensuring maximum stability for your little ones. Say goodbye to wobbling and hello to a secure and reliable potty experience! Discover the unparalleled excellence of this product, specially designed for the utmost comfort and well-being of your precious little ones.

- Introducing Splash Guards - the ultimate solution for a cleaner and more hygienic potty experience! Designed to direct the stream of urine, these innovative splash guards are specially crafted to cater to the needs of males. Say goodbye to messy accidents and hello to a hassle-free potty time. Plus, with the added bonus of preventing painful bumps, your little ones will be more comfortable than ever before. No more worries about needing to visit the potty again after an unfortunate mishap. Choose Splash Guards for a sanitary and stress-free potty experience! Experience the thrill of conquering new heights with our innovative Splash Safeguard Log! Say goodbye to the fear of falls as you confidently climb onto the log from your Potty chair. No more worries, just pure excitement! Introducing our revolutionary splash guards - now available with cushioned or detachable options! Experience the ultimate in protection and convenience with our state-of-the-art design. Say goodbye to messy splashes and hello to effortless maintenance. Upgrade your vehicle today with our premium splash guards! Introducing the ultimate solution for worry-free splashing! Ensure a comfortable fit with a generous inch of space between the splash guard and your little one's precious crotch.

- Introducing our innovative potty seat that guarantees maximum security! Our potty seat is designed to fasten securely to the potty chair, providing you with peace of mind and ensuring your child's safety. Discover the perfect grips.

- Introducing the Potty Dish - the ultimate solution for spill-free potty training! With its larger size, spills will be a thing of the past. Upgrade to the Potty Dish today and say goodbye to messy accidents! Introducing a dish that is effortlessly removable, allowing even the smallest of kids to empty them independently.

- Introducing the all-new Chair - experience the ultimate comfort and luxury of a soft, inviting potty chair. Say goodbye to chilly, hard seats and hello to a world of relaxation and convenience. Discover the ultimate in comfort with our selection of models featuring luxuriously padded chairs. Elevate your seating experience to new heights with our carefully curated collection.

- Introducing our revolutionary Potty seats with enhanced arm rests! Say goodbye to seat overturning mishaps. With our thoughtfully designed arm rests, children will instinctively grab hold and stay securely in place as they relax. Safety and comfort combined, for a worry-free potty experience.

- Introducing the revolutionary Stepping Stool! This incredible Potty Chair not only converts to a Potty Seat, but also helps you save money in the long run. Say goodbye to unnecessary expenses and hello to convenience and affordability!

- Introducing the incredible feature of portability! Imagine the convenience of having a potty chair that can easily collapse down for all your traveling needs. Say goodbye to bulky and cumbersome options, and say hello to the ultimate travel companion! Experience peace of mind with our sturdy hinges, designed to ensure that your device remains secure and stable even during the most demanding use.

- Discover the secret to potty training success with our revolutionary selection of potty seats and chairs. Watch as your child's resistance melts away and their curiosity is piqued by our carefully crafted designs. Say goodbye to rejection and hello to a potty training solution that truly captures their imagination.

Chapter 2

Introducing the Incredible Potty Chair Features!

Discover the essential features to consider when selecting your perfect potty chair.

Introducing the revolutionary Splash Guard! Say goodbye to messy spills and hello to clean countertops. With its innovative design, the Splash Guard keeps liquids contained, ensuring a hassle-free cooking experience.

Introducing the revolutionary Toddler Seat with Splash Safeguard, the ultimate solution for potty training boys! Say goodbye to messy accidents and hello to stress-free potty time. With its innovative design, this seat ensures that the potty sticks up, providing maximum comfort and convenience. Don't let potty training be a hassle any longer - choose the Toddler Seat with Splash Safeguard and make potty time a breeze! Introducing the ultimate splash safeguard for potty training young males - the revolutionary lip! Designed to provide maximum protection and support, this lip is a must-have for every parent. Say goodbye to messy accidents and hello to stress-free potty training. Get yours today!

Introducing the perfect solution for those adorable potty training mishaps! Say goodbye to those unexpected surprises on your floor when your little one is learning to use the potty. Our innovative product ensures that your son will master the art of positioning his "dangly piece" with ease. No more friendly fires to worry about!

Introducing the revolutionary splashguard, your ultimate solution for preventing any unwanted pee from escaping the potty. With its innovative design, it expertly bounces pee back into the bowl below, saving you from the hassle of cleaning up any mess. Say goodbye to those unpleasant accidents and hello to a cleaner, more hygienic experience.

Introducing the ultimate solution for hassle-free potty training! Say goodbye to messy accidents with our innovative splash guard. Designed with your convenience in mind, our splash guard is specifically crafted for females, ensuring a seamless and stress-free potty training experience. No more worries about unwanted splashes or messes. Trust our top-of-the-line splash guard to make potty training a breeze! Introducing a fascinating phenomenon: the subtle art of pelvic tilting while urinating, as observed in some girls. Prepare to be amazed by this intriguing display of bodily control. Introducing the revolutionary peeing position that will keep your floors pristine! Say goodbye to messy accidents with our Potty chair equipped with a state-of-the-art splash safeguard. No more splatters, no more worries!

Experience unwavering stability with our product.

Discover the ultimate solution for maintaining pristine floors - select a potty chair that boasts unbeatable stability, ensuring it remains steadfast and upright. Introducing the revolutionary Potty seat that guarantees your child's comfort and stability! Say goodbye to those embarrassing accidents caused by unstable seats. With our innovative design, your little one will confidently conquer the potty training journey without any mishaps. No more messy clean-ups or toppled seats - just pure progress and excitement. Invest in the best for your child's potty training success!

Discover the two key factors that determine the true ease of spilling a Potty:

- Weight - Discover the secret to effortless subject matter with our lightweight Potty. No more struggling with heavy burdens!

- Introducing the foundation of support - a revolutionary feature that ensures the Potty stays securely in place on your floor. Discover the secret to a spill-free Potty experience: the lower it touches the bottom, the more secure it becomes.

For optimal stability, ensure that the Potty is securely placed on the floor. Kneel down gracefully before it, and with utmost precision, position your hands on both sides of the Potty. Gently apply your weight, and with a seamless motion, shift one hand towards the other, maintaining perfect balance. Discover the ultimate Potty that surpasses all others with ease after careful evaluation.

Introducing the must-have feature for your tiles or wooden floor: a durable plastic lined bottom level. Say goodbye to worries and hello to peace of mind. Introducing our revolutionary plastic bottom that will put an end to the frustrating sliding and slipping of your Potty on your floor. Say goodbye to those precarious moments when your little one tries to climb aboard. Our innovative design ensures stability and peace of mind.

Discover the Wide Range of Stylish and Functional Potty Chairs

Allow your child to choose the Potty training chair or seat of their dreams. With a wide variety of playful and fun options available, it could be just the motivation your little one needs.

When it comes to Potty training, having the right equipment is absolutely crucial. Experience the ultimate sense of security and comfort while on the go, with easy access to the Potty. Experience the undeniable allure of embracing challenges and overcoming obstacles. The more arduous and demanding the journey, the less inclined they will be to resist it.

Discover the ultimate motivation for your child to master the art of using the bathroom - the perfect Potty seat! Make sure they have the right seat to embark on their potty training journey. Discover a wide array of vibrant colors, stylish designs, and innovative features in our collection of potty chairs, perfect for your little one's needs.

- Introducing our exquisite collection of Potty seats, designed to meet all your needs and preferences. Discover the perfect blend of style, comfort, and functionality with our wide range of options. From sleek and modern designs to charming and whimsical patterns, we have something to suit every taste.

- Introducing our innovative toddler Potty chair and travel Potty chairs. Say goodbye to messy accidents and hello to stress-free potty training!

Our toddler Potty chair is designed with your little one's comfort and independence in mind, making potty time a breeze. And for families on the go, our travel Potty chairs are the perfect solution to keep your child's potty routine consistent, no matter

- Introducing our exquisite collection of wooden Potty chairs. Crafted with precision and designed to perfection, these chairs are the epitome of style and functionality.

- Introducing our revolutionary musical Potty chairs!

- Introducing our revolutionary multifunctional potties!

- Introducing our exclusive line of personalized potty chairs.

Discover an extensive range of styles and colors to choose from. Experience the joy and enchantment of our delightful toddler Potty chairs. These charming and whimsical designs will bring a touch of magic to your little one's potty training journey.

Discover the perfect selection for your little one who adores princesses or cars. Delight their imagination with a captivating array of animals and vibrant colors. It's a truly fantastic choice! Discover these delightful chairs that resemble playful pets, with their whimsical shapes and vibrant shades of shiny pink and blue.

C h a p t e r   3

Discover the Art of Selecting the Perfect Potty

Discover the wide array of potties available in the market and let us guide you in selecting the perfect one for your needs. Discover the essential factors to consider when selecting the perfect potty before making your purchase.

Is your little one ready to take the leap from diapers? Experience the thrill of success! Introducing the ultimate purchase: the Potty, your new must-have item. Introducing our revolutionary approach to choosing the perfect Potty for your little one and your home. We have meticulously categorized the essential elements and crucial features to help you envision the ultimate Potty experience. Experience the ultimate convenience when shopping with your child. Whether she's interested or not, bring your son or daughter along for the trip. And if she's not, no worries! Simply take your tot's measurements before heading to the store. Shop with ease and style! Discover the essential factors to keep in mind.

Maximize Your Storage Potential

Introducing the world of potties, where convenience meets comfort. Prepare to be amazed by the two main types of potties that will revolutionize your potty training journey: the stand-alone potty and the seat reducer. Say goodbye to messy accidents and hello to a hassle-free experience! Introducing the ultimate stand-alone Potty that ticks all the boxes: security, size, and simplicity. When it comes to finding the perfect Potty, these three features are absolutely crucial. Say goodbye to worries and hello to peace of mind with our top-notch security. Experience the perfect fit with our carefully designed size. And enjoy effortless convenience with our user-friendly simplicity. Don't settle for less when it comes to your little one's comfort and safety. Choose our stand-alone Potty and make potty training a breeze. Introducing the ultimate Potty seat - designed for stability and comfort. Our innovative design ensures that your toddler's bottom fits snugly within the chair, providing a secure and comfortable experience. Plus, our Potty is incredibly user-friendly and a breeze to clean. Say goodbye to messy accidents and hello to hassle-free potty training with our top-of-the-line Potty seat.

 Introducing the incredible stand-alone Potty - the ultimate solution for your little one's potty training journey. Designed with your child in mind, this kid-size Potty allows them to gain independence by getting on and off all by themselves. No more waiting around for their turn, as this Potty ensures that your child will never monopolize it, especially in one-Potty households. Say goodbye to the hassle and hello to stress-free potty training with the stand-alone Potty. Introducing the incredible Potty, now available for free! With this amazing product, you can effortlessly showcase your Potty skills while simultaneously helping your younger child with their Potty training journey. Don't miss out on this opportunity - get your hands on the typical Potty today!

Introducing chair reducers, the ultimate solution for transforming any ordinary potty seat into a perfectly sized, kid-friendly throne. Experience the incredible benefits of these innovative accessories. Discover the incredible affordability of our space-saving Potty that is not only cost-effective but also takes up minimal living area. Introducing the revolutionary Typical Potty for your little one! Say goodbye to messy transitions from stand-alone Potty to adult Potty. With our innovative design, your child will effortlessly adapt to the Typical Potty, making cleanup a breeze. Experience the convenience and cleanliness like never before! Introducing chair reducers - the perfect solution for kids who love to imitate! These incredible accessories are not only practical, but also a great fit for little ones who want to mimic the grown-ups. Introducing the ultimate source of inspiration for young ones who aspire to follow in the footsteps of their older siblings, cousins, or friends - they are the perfect motivators! Keep in mind that selecting a chair reducer can be a game-changer. By opting for a stool, you can assist your child in effortlessly transitioning to the Potty. Not only does it provide ample foot support, but it also aids in the process of expelling pee or poop. Make the right choice for your little one's comfort and convenience.

Introducing the latest innovation in potty training essentials - our stand-alone potties and chair reducers! Designed with your child's comfort in mind, these incredible products come equipped with convenient handles. Not only do these handles provide added support, but they also help your little one feel more at ease during this important milestone. Introducing an exciting new way for kids to experience the thrill of transportation! Our innovative product provides them with a means to drive and explore, all while having a blast. Say goodbye to boredom and hello to endless fun! Introducing chair reducers - the ultimate solution for effortless chair management. With our innovative handles, you can effortlessly retrieve your chair and stow it away with ease. Say goodbye to clutter and hello to convenient storage options. Experience the convenience of chair reducers today! Still unsure about what your child will prefer? Choose a multitasking Potty that can effortlessly handle various tasks while saving valuable space. Introducing the incredible world of stand-alone potties! These innovative potties come equipped with detachable seats that can be used as a chair reducer or a Potty seat. But that's not all - these potties also feature convenient shut lids that can double as stools. Experience the ultimate in versatility and functionality with our stand-alone potties!

Discover the Perfect Fit and Size for Your Potty Needs

Discover a wide variety of potties available in various quantities and rim sizes, ensuring that you select the perfect one with an impeccable fit. Experience ultimate comfort and support for your toddler with our innovative chair design. Say goodbye to uncomfortable and stressful seating experiences. Our chair ensures that your little one's bottom level is perfectly draped and nestled within the rim, providing unparalleled comfort and relaxation. Trust us to create a seating solution that will keep your toddler happy and content. Discover the perfect chair size that will provide your child with ultimate comfort and stability. Ensure their little bottoms are perfectly aligned, resting effortlessly on the chair, while their feet find a secure place on the floor or stool.

Discover the ultimate solution for protecting your vehicle from unwanted splashes and debris - Splash Guards! Don't let dirt, mud, or rocks ruin the pristine appearance of your car. With our top-of-the-line Splash Guards, you can say goodbye to

Discover the secret to minimizing post-potty cleanup when potty training your little one - the chair with a splash guard. Say goodbye to messy accidents and hello to hassle-free training! Discover the perfect potty seat that strikes the ideal balance - one that's tall enough to prevent any accidents, yet low enough for your little one to comfortably sit on their own.

Discover the Excitement of Extra Fun Features

Discover a world of potties that go beyond the ordinary. With a wide range of captivating themes, enchanting lamps, delightful songs, and captivating sound files, these potties are designed to make potty time an extraordinary experience. But the question remains: are they truly worth it? Introducing an exciting new experience that is sure to captivate your child's imagination! Imagine the joy on your little one's face as they discover the thrilling competition car flushing sound or unlock the magical wand reward track on the Potty. This is an opportunity that will truly ignite their interest and keep them engaged for hours on end. Discover the true essence of it all, Discover the art of parenting Experience the true joy of parenting by giving your child the ultimate delight - your heartfelt compliment. No flashy light show, sticker, or tiny candy can compare to the joy it brings. Get ready to applaud, give a warm embrace, or bust out a special dance to celebrate your child's achievements, and leave the electronics behind.

Experience the convenience of Easy Emptying.

Introducing our revolutionary stand-alone Potty! Say goodbye to the hassle of extra dirty work. With our innovative design, you'll experience a whole new level of convenience and cleanliness. Discover the power of checking the box's outside or browsing online product critiques to unveil the secrets of effortlessly emptying and cleaning the container. Introducing an array of toilet models, each with its own unique installation process.

Some boast a simple and hassle-free two-step procedure, ensuring a seamless experience. However, there are others that may demand a bit more effort, necessitating the disassembly of half the toilet on each occasion. Choose wisely to find the perfect fit for your needs.

Discover the Magic of Potty Training in Just One Day!

Experience the greatness for yourself!

Or is it simply too good to be true?

Discover the power of perspective and the art of managing expectations.

Introducing a revolutionary technique that's not just another ordinary solution. It's not a magic pill, but rather a powerful tool that, when combined with careful planning, meticulous preparation, and unwavering determination, has the potential to unlock your true potential and help you thrive in any endeavor you set your mind to.

Experience the transformative power of dedication and determination as you embark on a journey towards success. Embrace the challenges that come your way, including the occasional mishap, and take charge of cleaning up any unexpected accidents. With your unwavering commitment, nothing can stand in your way. Discover the transformative power of learning from mistakes. Embrace the fact that your child will grow and thrive, just like the rest of us.

Discover the remarkable effectiveness of this method that has proven successful for countless parents. Experience the extraordinary with our exclusive "BIG DAY" package. Make every moment count on this special occasion. Experience the ultimate milestone as your child embarks on a journey of true potty training. Say goodbye to diapers and welcome the era of "big kid" Potty training pants.

Master the Art of Potty Training

Introducing the key to a truly fulfilling and triumphant

"BIG DAY" - the art of dedicating your time to preparation and planning. Embrace the alternative activities that life has to offer and unlock the secret to a truly satisfying experience. Experience the effortless efficiency of our streamlined process, where the appearance and planning can be completed in just one hour. The duration may vary depending on your level of preparedness and the needs of your child. Trust us to make this journey as smooth and stress-free as possible. Discover the perfect amount of time to prepare for the "BIG DAY" - it all depends on your child. Discover the fascinating world of children's needs. While some children may sail smoothly through life, others may benefit from a little extra attention. Explore the possibilities of follow-up and unlock the potential for growth and development.

Introducing Potty Trained in One Day - the ultimate solution to your potty training woes!

Discover the ultimate solution for potty training your child! Say goodbye to diapers as your son or daughter embarks on a journey to master the art of using the potty.

Watch as they learn to effortlessly pee in the potty and understand the importance of this milestone. Get ready for a hassle-free potty training experience!

Imagine a day where everything runs smoothly, where you effortlessly glide through your tasks and responsibilities. But here's the secret: it all starts with careful preparation. You, my friend, hold the power to make this happen. By gathering all the necessary items and organizing your child and yourself, you are already taking the first steps towards a successful day. And guess what? You're already on the right track by reading this book. So keep going, because greatness awaits you. Prepare yourself both mentally and physically to handle potty incidents and the subsequent clean-ups resulting from these accidents. After a long and eventful day, it's time to tackle the task of tidying up any unexpected potty accidents. But don't worry, we've got you covered. In addition to that, it's important to have a follow-up conversation with your little one to ensure they understand your expectations crystal clear.

Discover the incredible speed at which young children

learn with this revolutionary system. Prepare to be amazed as potty incidents become a thing of the past in just a matter of days. Introducing our remarkable solution for parents: a week-long journey of incident-free bliss for most children. But wait, there's more! For those exceptional little ones who crave excitement, we offer a thrilling 14-day adventure filled with the possibility of mishaps. Choose the experience that suits your child's unique spirit!

Experience the power of persistence and witness a worry-free environment for you and your child in just two weeks or less! Introducing a revolutionary solution that will make you forget all about diapers or pull-ups! Say goodbye to the hassle and inconvenience with our game-changing product.

Still not convinced? Discover the incredible results that the Potty Trained in One Day technique has achieved for countless other parents.

Discover the Ultimate Guide to Potty Training Success in Just 24 Hours!

Discover the revolutionary technique outlined in the Parent's Potty Training Guide: How to Potty Train within a Day, where success hinges on the mastery of two fundamental concepts:

Discover the power of teaching as the ultimate method to truly comprehend any subject. At our company, we understand the power of visual and auditory learning for children. Discover the fascinating world of learning as these remarkable beings absorb actions and behaviors, effortlessly mirroring the things they have keenly observed. Discover the ultimate solution for teaching your child proper Potty training behavior - a doll! There's nothing quite like the power of a doll to demonstrate the right way to use the toilet. Say goodbye to messy accidents and hello to successful potty training with our incredible doll model.

Introducing the all-new, revolutionary "•"! Experience a product like no other, designed to exceed your expectations and enhanceIntroducing a groundbreaking concept that revolves around the undeniable truth that behavior is intricately molded by consequence. Discover the power of parental influence as children learn and grow from the consequences of their actions. Tap into this invaluable parenting tool that you've undoubtedly utilized to great effect.

Discover the undeniable appeal of both logical and natural consequences. Experience the authentic outcomes of your child's own endeavors. Discover the power of logical email address details, a reflection of behavior that is often instilled by parents.

Introducing Potty Scotty or Potty Patty, the ultimate Potty training doll designed to help your child master the art of using the toilet. With your guidance and the help of this anatomically correct doll, your little one will learn all the essential "heading Potty" behaviors in no time. Introducing your child to the wonderful world of potty training! As they embark on this exciting journey, they will soon realize that the simple act of consuming leads to the natural urge to urinate. And what awaits them after successfully using the potty? A delightful array of rewards! From heartfelt words of praise to delightful treats, engaging toys, and even a grand celebration with a

Potty party. Get ready to celebrate each milestone with joy and excitement!

Experience the revolutionary method of effortlessly guiding Scotty to the Potty!

Introducing our revolutionary doll training system! Watch as your little one learns the valuable lesson of not using the potty through the natural consequence of wet underwear. Say goodbye to messy accidents and hello to potty success! Experience the transformative power of our innovative training method that effortlessly guides your little one towards the path of success. Say goodbye to undesired behavior and hello to a future filled with potty training triumphs. Discover the secret to forward progress today!

Discover just how effortless it truly is. Experience the incredible power of this revolutionary product - it works like magic!

Discover the secret to success: preparation and planning. Just like in life, achievement is the result of careful preparation and strategic planning. Introducing the undeniable truth: there is no miracle pill. Achieving your goals requires dedication, hard work, and unwavering determination. It's time to unleash your inner strength and embark on a journey of self-improvement.

Discover the ultimate guide to effortlessly guiding your child's journey with this remarkable book. Unveiling the secrets of effective parenting, this invaluable resource provides you with a detailed, step-by-step approach to nurturing your child's development.

Experience stress-free potty training and enjoy a worry-free trip!

Experience a remarkable transformation in your surroundings, brought about by a vacation or other travel, which can often lead to common challenges with potty training in children.

Introducing our revolutionary travel programs designed to ensure your child's comfort and well-being every step of the way. Say goodbye to the stress and mishaps caused by unfamiliar potties, as our expertly crafted itineraries prioritize your child's needs. No more worries about constipation ruining your trip. Choose our travel programs for a seamless and worry-free experience.

Experience the power of positive change! While some responses may be short-term and fade away as your child adjusts to the new schedule or returns to the old one, there are instances where certain behaviors can take hold. These behaviors, like withholding stool or delaying urination, may require weeks or even a couple of months to correct. But fear not, with patience and the right approach, lasting solutions are within reach!

Introducing the ultimate solution to all your potty-related travel woes! Say goodbye to those pesky problems and hello to a seamless potty experience for your little one. It's simple - just keep their potty routine while traveling as close to their regular routine at home as humanly possible. Trust us, you won't want to leave home without it!

Planning a car vacation? Don't forget to bring your kid's very own Potty or opt for a convenient travel potty.

Ensure a stress-free journey for the whole family!

Introducing the ultimate travel hack for parents! Before you embark on your next flight, make sure to whisk your little one to the Potty at the international airport. But wait, there's more! Don't forget to pack their beloved stuffed animals or cherished items to transform any public or hotel Potty into a cozy and familiar oasis. Say goodbye to those scary moments and hello to stress-free travels!

Experience the joy of guiding your child on their potty journey and be prepared to provide even more encouragement than if you were not traveling.

Chapter 4

Discover the Incredible Benefits and Drawbacks of the Revolutionary Potty Chair/Seat!

Prepare to be amazed! Discover the perfect moment to embark on the exciting journey of potty training your precious little one! Discover the ultimate secret to stress-free potty training! With the help of a top-notch potty, you can conquer this challenging milestone with ease. Say goodbye to frustration and hello to success!

Introducing an extensive array of potties available on the market, finding the perfect one can be quite a daunting challenge. But worry not, we've got you covered! Introducing the ultimate guide that will revolutionize your understanding - from the moment you start reading until the very end. Discover the hidden talent within you as a Potty Equipment Expert. Experience the ultimate coolness, right before your eyes!

The Potty Chair - Revolutionize Your Child's Potty

Training Journey!

Introducing our latest innovation: a product that is not only low to the ground, but also incredibly easy for your son or daughter to use all on their own. Say goodbye to any struggles or frustrations - this is the ultimate solution you've been waiting for. Discover the perfect starting point for any parent embarking on the journey of potty training their child - a reliable and practical potty seat.

Experience the adorable and heartwarming sight of a baby sitting confidently on the Potty chair, with their pants down. Witness this precious moment of independence and growth as they embark on their potty training journey.

Introducing the remarkable Potty Chair - a small chair designed to revolutionize your potty training journey. With its innovative design, this chair sits gracefully on the floor, boasting a recessed area meticulously crafted to capture every drop of pee and poop. Say goodbye to messy accidents and hello to a stress-free potty experience! Experience ultimate comfort for your son or daughter with our low elevation design, allowing them to relax with their feet gently touching the ground.

Introducing our revolutionary potty seat that will make your life easier! Say goodbye to the hassle of cleaning up after your child's bathroom breaks. With our innovative design, all you have to do is effortlessly dispose of the waste and effortlessly rinse it away in the sink. No more mess, no more stress. Experience the convenience and cleanliness you deserve with our state-of-the-art potty seat.

Discover the convenience of portable potty chairs. Introducing the revolutionary Potty seat that goes wherever you go! With its portable design, you can now ensure that your child always has access to a Potty, no matter which room they're in. Say goodbye to inconvenient bathroom trips and hello to ultimate convenience!

Experience the many advantages of our product:

- Transform any room in your house with ease.

- Provide your child with unparalleled comfort as their feet rest effortlessly on the floor.

- Experience the thrill of starting from the top with no fear of falling. Reach new heights without worrying about the consequences. Embrace the freedom of limitless possibilities.

- Introducing our revolutionary product that makes it effortless for your son or daughter to comfortably lay down, all on their own. No more need for your constant assistance!

Introducing the drawbacks:

- Requires cleaning after each use.

- Introducing the ultimate solution for teaching your son or daughter the art of using a regular Potty!

- Introducing our revolutionary toddler seat with an adjustable height feature! Say goodbye to uncomfortable seating for taller toddlers. With our innovative design, you can easily adjust the seat height to ensure the perfect fit for your little one.

No more compromises when it comes to comfort and convenience. Upgrade to our toddler seat today and give your child the seating experience they deserve.

Discover the Ultimate Selection of Potty Chairs.

Discover an array of exquisite Potty chairs that are sure to captivate your attention. Let's delve into the fascinating details of each one:

- Introducing the revolutionary Single Piece Potty Chair - the ultimate solution for your little one's potty training needs. Say goodbye to messy accidents and hello to hassle-free potty time!

- Introducing our exquisite Traditional Solitary Piece Potty Chair.

- Introducing the ultimate solution for potty training - the Two-Piece Potty Chair! Say goodbye to messy accidents and hello to stress-free potty time. With its innovative design and top-notch quality, this potty chair is a game-changer. Get ready to make potty

- Introducing the Deluxe Potty Chair - the ultimate solution for your potty training needs. Say goodbye to messy accidents and hello to a comfortable and convenient potty experience. With its sleek design and top-notch features, this potty chair is a must-have for every parent.

Introducing the extraordinary world of potty chairs, where innovation meets convenience. Crafted with utmost care, our potty chairs are made from a single, meticulously molded piece of high-quality plastic. Experience the epitome of comfort and durability with our exceptional range of potty chairs. Introducing our revolutionary Potty seat that not only gets the job done, but does so with unparalleled comfort and ease of cleaning. Say goodbye to unpleasant experiences and heavy maintenance. Upgrade to our innovative Potty seat today!

Introducing the ultimate solution for potty training - our Two-Piece Potty Chair with a convenient removable insert. Say goodbye to messy accidents and hello to stress-free potty time!

Epitome of modern potty chairs

A true game-changer in the world of potty training. Say goodbye to ordinary and embrace the extraordinary with our exceptional line of potty chairs. Introducing the incredible Potty Chair Deluxe, a revolutionary product that lives up to its name by offering not just one, but two separate items!

Introducing our revolutionary product: the ultimate seating solution for your little one! Our outer plastic seat provides unparalleled support and comfort, ensuring your child's utmost satisfaction while sitting. But that's not all - our innovative design also includes an inner plastic bowl that effortlessly captures and contains your baby's waste, making cleanup a breeze. Say goodbye to messy accidents and hello to convenience and peace of mind. Invest in the future of parenting with our cutting-edge seat and bowl combo.

Make cleanup a breeze after your child is finished with

our Potty Chair. Simply remove the inner bucket and give it a quick clean before returning it. It's that easy! Discover the effortless convenience of cleaning a detachable insert, making it a breeze compared to the hassle of cleaning the entire Potty chair in your kitchen sink.

Deluxe Potty Chair

The ultimate solution for your little one's potty training journey. This top-of-the-line potty chair is designed with utmost comfort and convenience in mind. Say goodbye

Introducing the Deluxe Potty Seat - the ultimate solution for all your potty training needs! Experience a world of incredible benefits with this revolutionary product:

Introducing our revolutionary storage solution! With our innovative hooks and grab drawers, you can now keep your paper or baby wipes conveniently nearby and easily accessible for those crucial moments when your little one has completed their business. Say goodbye to fumbling around for supplies and hello to a more organized and efficient diaper changing experience!

Introducing our innovative solution for potty training - the Lights and Noises potty! Say goodbye to boring bathroom routines and hello to excitement and motivation. When your child is done with their business, they can simply press the lever and be rewarded with a delightful flushing audio and eye-catching flashing lights. Make potty time a fun and rewarding experience for your little one! Introducing the incredible potty chair that goes above and beyond! Not only does it provide a comfortable seat for your child, but it also features a delightful musical surprise. Imagine the joy on your little one's face as they sit down and are greeted with their favorite tunes. Make potty time a fun and enjoyable experience with our innovative potty chair. Get yours today!

Introducing our revolutionary Deodorizer - the ultimate solution to eliminate any unpleasant odors caused by your baby's poop. Say goodbye to those embarrassing moments when your house is filled with unwanted smells before you even have a chance to clean the Potty. With our Deodorizer, you can enjoy a fresh and odor-free environment, ensuring a pleasant experience for both you and your little one.

Introducing our luxurious Cushioned Chair - the perfect throne for your little one to conquer their tasks in utmost comfort and style. Crafted with an incredibly smooth surface, this chair provides the ideal space for your child to accomplish their business with ease.

Introducing the My Fun Sticker Potty - the potty chair that comes with a delightful surprise! Experience the joy of stickers with our specially designed potty chairs. Each chair is adorned with a band of stickers, adding a touch of fun and excitement to your little one's potty training journey. Introducing our incredible stickers that give your child the power to create their very own one-of-a-kind Potty experience.

Introducing the revolutionary iPad stand - because we take your needs seriously. Introducing the ultimate potty experience - now with an iPad tablet! Watch as your child's imagination soars while they conquer the potty training journey. Say goodbye to boredom and hello to endless entertainment. It's time to turn potty time into playtime!

Introducing the incredible Deluxe Potty seats - the ultimate solution to your potty training woes! These seats are a true catch-22, offering a plethora of amazing features that are guaranteed to make potty training a breeze for your little one. Say goodbye to the struggles and hello to success with Deluxe Potty seats! On the flipside, every additional feature contributes to the Potty's enhanced functionality. However, it's important to note that these features also increase its weight, which means that cleaning becomes a necessary task when it inevitably comes into contact with urine or feces (a very real possibility).

The revolutionary Multifunction Potty Chair

The ultimate solution for potty training success! This innovative chair is designed to make the potty training journey a breeze for both parents and little ones.

Introducing the revolutionary multifunction potty seat, designed to seamlessly grow alongside your child. Introducing an exquisite collection of multifunction Potty chairs, designed to meet all your needs and more. Discover the perfect blend of style and functionality with our wide range of mixtures, carefully crafted to provide the ultimate convenience for you and your little one. Experience the epitome of versatility with our exceptional selection of Potty chairs, tailored to make potty training a breeze. Explore the possibilities and choose the ideal combination that suits your unique requirements.

Introducing the revolutionary 2-in-1 Potty Seat! Experience the ultimate convenience with a removable Potty seat that will change the way you potty train your little one. Say goodbye to messy clean-ups and hello to a hassle-free potty training experience!

Introducing the incredible 3-in-1 Potty Chair - the ultimate solution for your little one's potty training journey! This innovative product combines the functionality of a potty chair, a potty chair, and a step-stool, all in one convenient design. Say goodbye to clutter and hello to simplicity with this versatile and space-saving solution. Get ready to make potty training a breeze with the 3-in-1 Potty Chair!

Introducing the incredible 4-in-1 Potty Chair! This versatile product is not just a potty chair, but also a step-stool and storage solution all in one. With its innovative design, you'll have everything you need conveniently at your fingertips. Say goodbye to clutter and hello to convenience with the 4-in-1 Potty Chair!

Introducing the extraordinary Bravo 3-in-1 Potty, the ultimate combination Potty chair that sets the standard for excellence. Prepare to be amazed by its versatility and functionality. Say goodbye to multiple potty seats cluttering your bathroom, because the Bravo 3-in-1 Potty is here to revolutionize your potty training experience. Get ready for a whole new level of convenience and innovation!

Indulge in the ultimate experience with a delightful fusion of baby equipment. Unlock the power of versatility! Instead of excelling at just one task, imagine being proficient in multiple areas. Embrace the beauty of being a well-rounded individual. Discover the secret to a stress-free experience by choosing to purchase your solutions separately, rather than opting for a seemingly cheap all-in-one solution. By taking this approach, you can ensure that you are setting yourself up for success and avoiding unnecessary hassle.

Introducing the all-new mixture potties - the perfect solution for your little one's potty training needs! However, it's important to note that one downside of these innovative potties is that they come with a few more parts than traditional options. But fear not, as the benefits far outweigh this minor inconvenience. Get ready to embark on a hassle-free potty training journey with our top-of-the-line mixture potties! Experience the freedom to spend quality time with your baby, while we take care of the cleaning. Say goodbye to the hassle of cleaning multiple items and say hello to more precious moments with your little one.

Methods for Handling Potty Training

Regression

Your potty-trained youngster is having accidents all of a sudden? Discover the cause of Potty regression and take steps to stop it.

Everything is going well; it appears that your child has mastered potty training, so you think you can finally say goodbye to diapers. But then all of a sudden he starts getting into catastrophes again, and you wonder what went wrong. We'll explain why kids frequently regress in their potty training efforts and offer advice on how to proceed.

Verify if it is a true regression.

Rest assured that most children undergo regression in their potty training; this is a perfectly typical occurrence. However, question if your child was actually potty trained in the first place. While occasional failures are normal throughout the initial days, weeks, and even months of potty training, keep in mind that a potty-trained child should want to be near the potty. Therefore, a child who experiences numerous instances every day and doesn't seem to value them shouldn't be considered "potty trained." Thus, think about if your child was ready for potty training; if so, seek for strategies to go back on the correct track; if not, ask your pediatrician when she/he believes your child may be ready.

Avoid Overreacting

Don't express disappointment if your child has an accident; doing so may make your child even more apprehensive, which may then result in further potty issues. Reverting to diapers can help ease the frustration that comes with potty training relapse, but try not to lose hope. If your child is dry out when you check, give them a round of applause. "Oops, you'd a crash, let's go lay on the potty" and proceed without passing judgment if he or she isn't. Remember to stay positive rather than reprimand or yell at your child. You want your kids to appear confident rather than fear punishment should they make a mistake.

Taking Care of the Main Reasons for Regression

If you don't solve the entire issue, you won't be able to

avoid the setbacks. Look for the cause of the regression and try to help the child go back to where they were by addressing it. From both the director of a child study center and your department in developmental and behavioral pediatrics at the University of Oklahoma Health Sciences Middle. For example, a lot of kids start experiencing stressful life transitions during times when things are changing, like moving to a new college or getting a new sibling. Your child may become proficient at potty training again once your lives settle down, but even if she manages to get through the day without any accidents, she might still have accidents at night. Many children who are dry during the daytime hours are not dry at night for extended periods of time. Control during the day is not the same as control during the night and during naps. Potty training regression can also be caused by medical conditions, and constipation is a prevalent one. If a child has trouble using the potty, they may use it exclusively to avoid pushing and straining themselves. Make sure your child drinks enough of water and soluble fiber, but if she's afraid to use the potty, make it more pleasant for her by reading stories or playing entertaining video games while she's sleeping.

Accidents frequently occur when a child is having too much fun playing or doing a task and doesn't want to stop, presumably to use the potty. To resolve this scenario, tell your child that she is "an enormous lady" even though it is natural to occasionally ignore the potty. Next, lead her to the bathroom every few hours at home, and ask her teachers to see to it that she uses the restroom often. A youngster can be redirected back on the correct path with some gentle, straightforward encouragement and reminders to use the potty. Urge your child to try using the potty when she wakes up, before eating, before going to bed, and right before leaving the house.

Acknowledgements

Behold the magnificent triumph of this extraordinary book, a testament to the divine intervention of God Almighty and the unwavering love and support of my cherished Family, devoted Fans, avid Readers, loyal Customers, and dear Friends. Their ceaseless encouragement has paved the way for this resounding success.

www.ingramcontent.com/pod-product-compliance
Lightning Source LLC
Chambersburg PA
CBHW031133020426
42333CB00012B/362